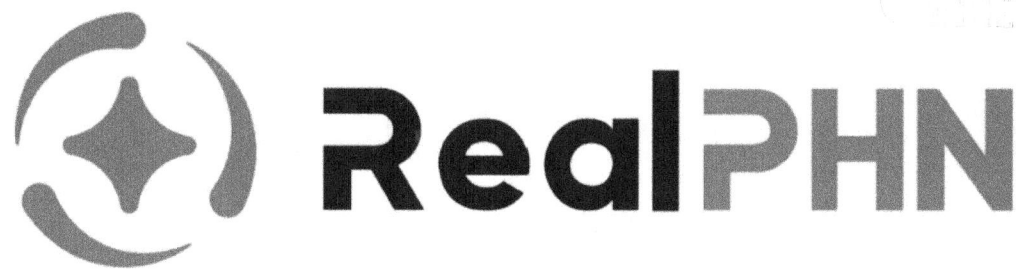

Real Population Health™

"What the Heck" is Happening with US Healthcare 2023?

Rural Healthcare Appendix

Harry Spring

Copyright © 2024 by Harry Spring
All rights reserved.

> **Introductory Position**
> US Rural healthcare's circumstances and challenges present-
>
> *MAJOR POSITIVE NATIONAL OPPORTUNITIES!!*
>
> Rural US
> 18,723 communities under 50,000 people
> 46,000,000 people.
> All very different in numerous ways.
> Common need? Better health, better healthcare, lower cost.
>
> An important rural appendix to
> "What the Heck" is happening with US Healthcare 2023

Contents

Why the Rural Healthcare Appendix to the Original *"What the Heck" is Happening in US Healthcare 2023?* v

Executive summary vii

Section 1 The foundation viii
Section 2 Healthcare's operating structure on its foundation 4
Section 3 "What the heck" is happening with Healthcare 2023? 8
Section 4 A proven healthcare improvement process 11
Section 5 A template for US healthcare 16

Summary 21
Rural Healthcare Appendix 21
About the Author 27

Why the Rural Healthcare Appendix to the Original *"What the Heck" is Happening in US Healthcare 2023?*

Six generalizations determine <u>rural healthcare</u> **MUST** have its own focus.

1. 97% of US land is rural.
2. 15% of population 46 million live in rural US, larger than any single US state.
3. 90% of the food we eat, grown in rural US.
4. 17.5% rural over age 65 compared to 13.8% urban or 27% higher rate.
5. 42% "of Americans would like to live in rural areas or towns."
6. Approx 2,000 hospitals, 30% "teetering on the edge of closure."

Data source URLs are in the rural appendix.

Real Population Health success hinges on two integral fundamentals:

1. Relationships amongst individuals, health focused health professionals (Personal Health Nurses and Primary Care Doctors/NP's/PA's).
2. Data, information, and deployment supporting ongoing relationships.

Rural US is perfectly positioned and pressured into deploying those Real Population Health fundamentals.

Those positions set the structures for the Rural US appendix to "What the Heck" is happening with US HealthCare 2023.

1. The index introduction on this page.
2. The original book *"What the Heck" is Happening with US Healthcare 2023?*
3. The Rural Healthcare appendix describing rural US, rural healthcare, and opportunities for achieving Real Population Health™ for residents in rural US.

The material provides readers with enhanced understanding of data/information supporting individuals in their pursuits of better health, healthcare, and cost.

Rural Healthcare Appendix fits within the broader Real Population Health offerings, all on Amazon/Kindle including:

- *Real Population Health™ Operating Manual 2022*, providing details of how to build, operate, and deliver better health, healthcare, and cost.
- A companion work about data/information management in appendix form similar to this.
- Eight brief Real Population Health™ handbooks for each stakeholder.

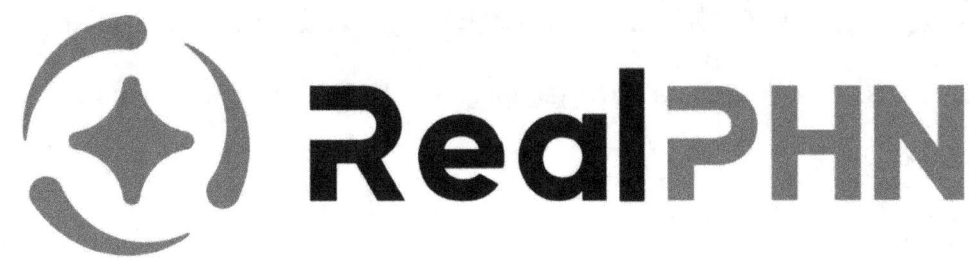

Real Population Health™

"What the Heck" is Happening with US Healthcare 2023?

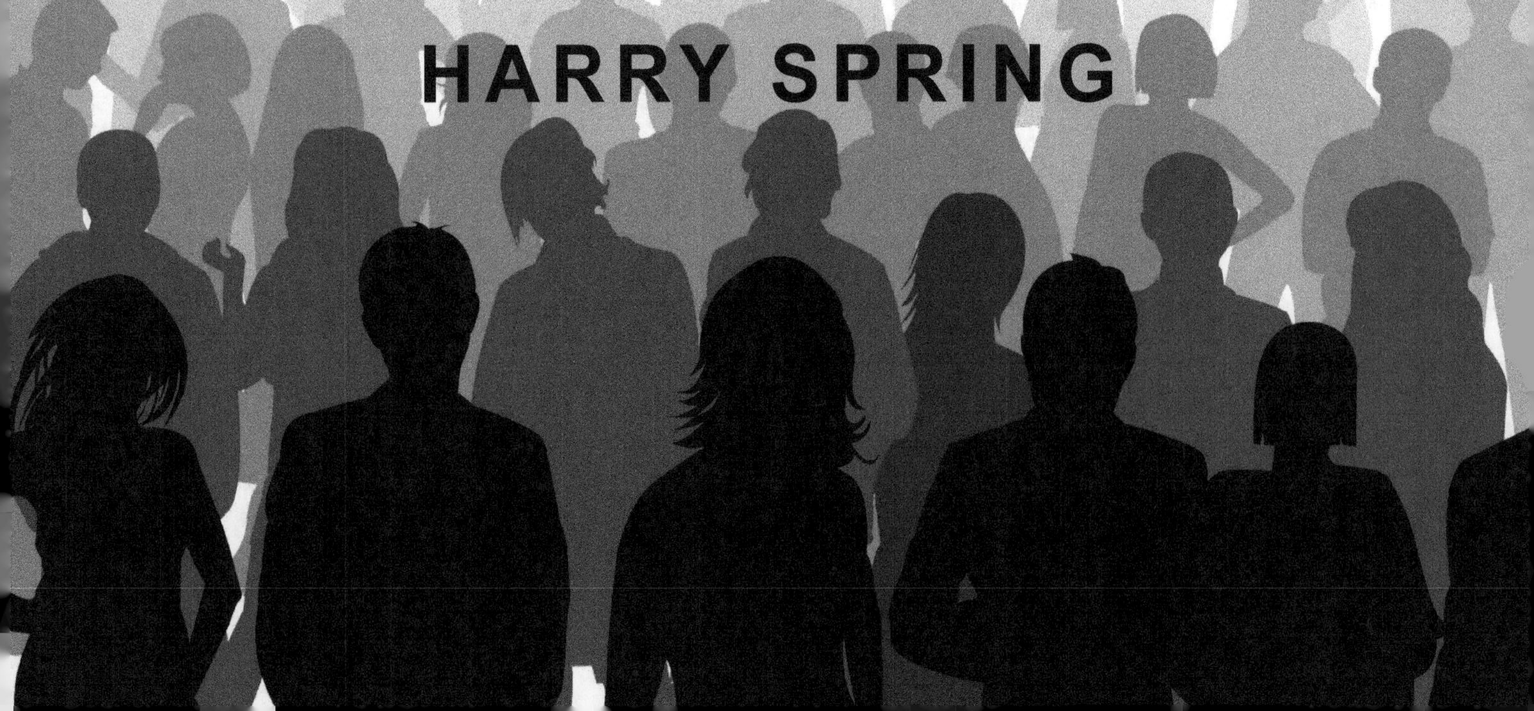

HARRY SPRING

Executive summary

In one visual, Diagram 1 shows "What the heck" is going on with US healthcare.

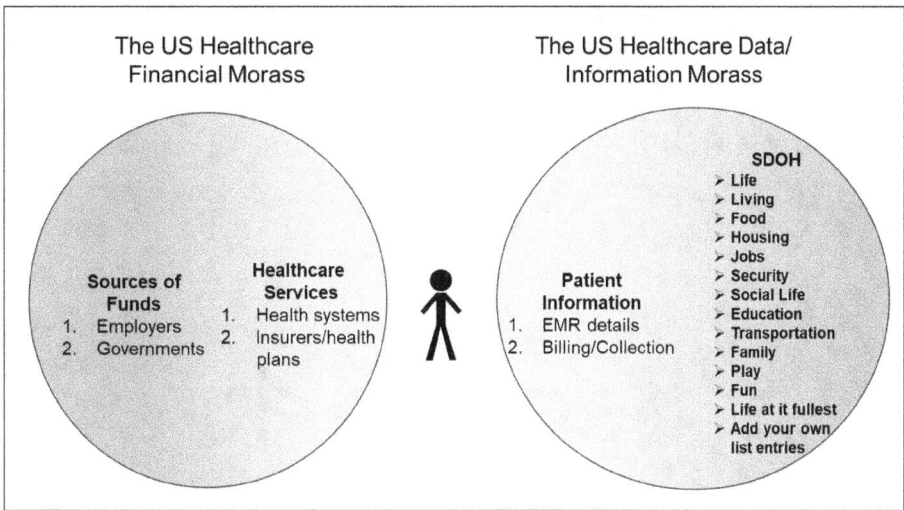

The financial morass

1. Individuals and consumers are caught in the middle of an annual four-trillion-dollar medical treatment healthcare system.
2. Employers and governments foot the bill.
3. Health systems deliver the services.
4. Individual consumers get caught in all the contracts, networks, billing, adjustments, transparency, etc. They just want to get well.

The data/information morass

1. Most stored data are medical treatment focused.
2. 80% of health problems are related to social determinants of health (SDOH).

The current system clearly doesn't work! But what can be done?

The solution? A proven healthcare improvement process?

> 1. **Creative use of data and information** that are individual and population specific.
>
> 2. **Creating and operating "relationships"** amongst individuals, their SDOH information, a person such as a Personal Health Nurse™ and needed resources.

In many ways, it's just that simple. In real life? Close to impossible.

Section 1:
The foundation

The beginning

A merican healthcare is broken. And American healthcare systems must transform radically to lead the repair.

Hospitals Need to Focus on Social Drivers of American Health | Time

There is broad acceptance of "health care is broken."
Regardless of politics and other forces,
there is general agreement.
We need to do better.
We need to do things differently.

Nearly all the money we spend on healthcare goes for medical interventions. However, clinical care is responsible for at most 20% of health outcomes.

Hospitals Need to Focus on Social Drivers of American Health | Time

These statements are public, national, and widely agreed upon.

This book is written in these beginning contexts for three reasons:

1. The healthcare system is really broken and operating on a **fundamentally flawed foundation**.

2. There are historical and current actions taken by various healthcare stakeholders that improve the system and deliver triple aim results: a) better health, b) better healthcare, and c) better (lower) cost. The actions can be replicated with positive results.

3. Within current foundations, structures, and operations, there is a consistent, historical, and currently **proven healthcare improvement process** that any of healthcare's six stakeholders can lead.

Diagram 2: US healthcare's fundamentally flawed foundation

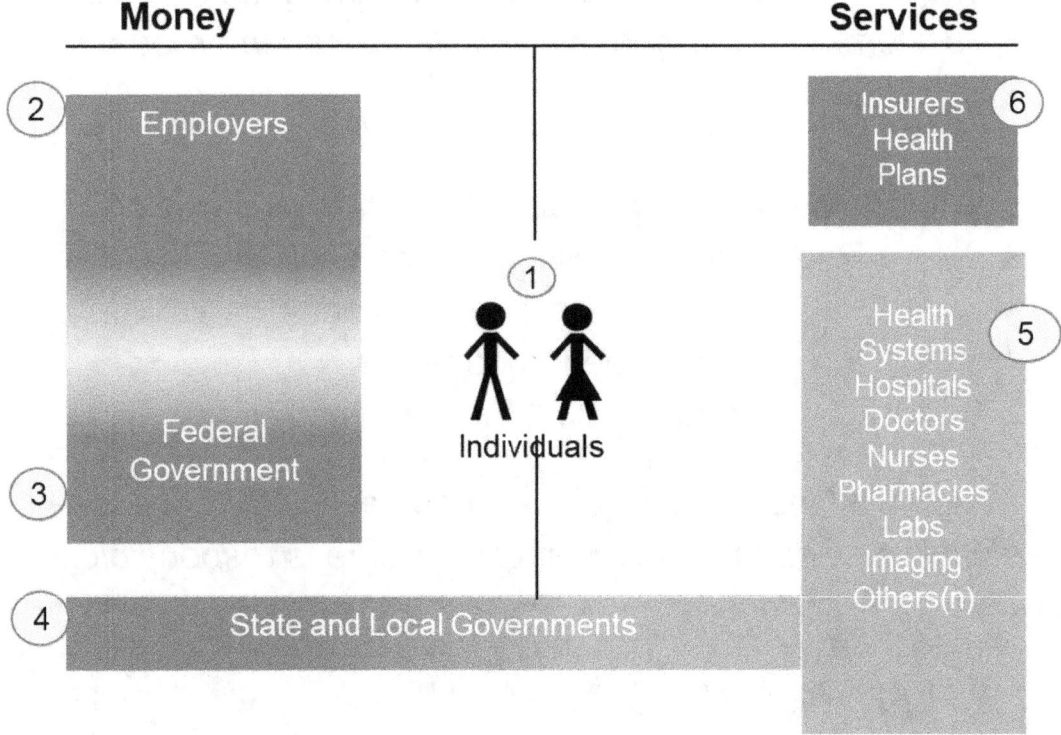

Generally, there are six healthcare stakeholders.

- **Individuals** are healthcare's consumers/patients. 80% of the time they're not patients. Where do they belong then?
- Funding, payment, and money come from **employers** and **governments**.
- **Health systems** provide healthcare/medical treatment services.
- **Insurers** and **health plans** contract with health systems and administer the contracts and reimbursement.

Diagram 2 shows that healthcare financing is win-lose. When individuals are healthy and productive, healthcare loses. When people are sick and injured, healthcare wins while employers and governments lose through plan cost increases.

The logical conclusion? *American healthcare is broken.*

Something must be and can be done through proven healthcare improvement models.

Diagram 3: US Healthcare's flawed foundation with operations

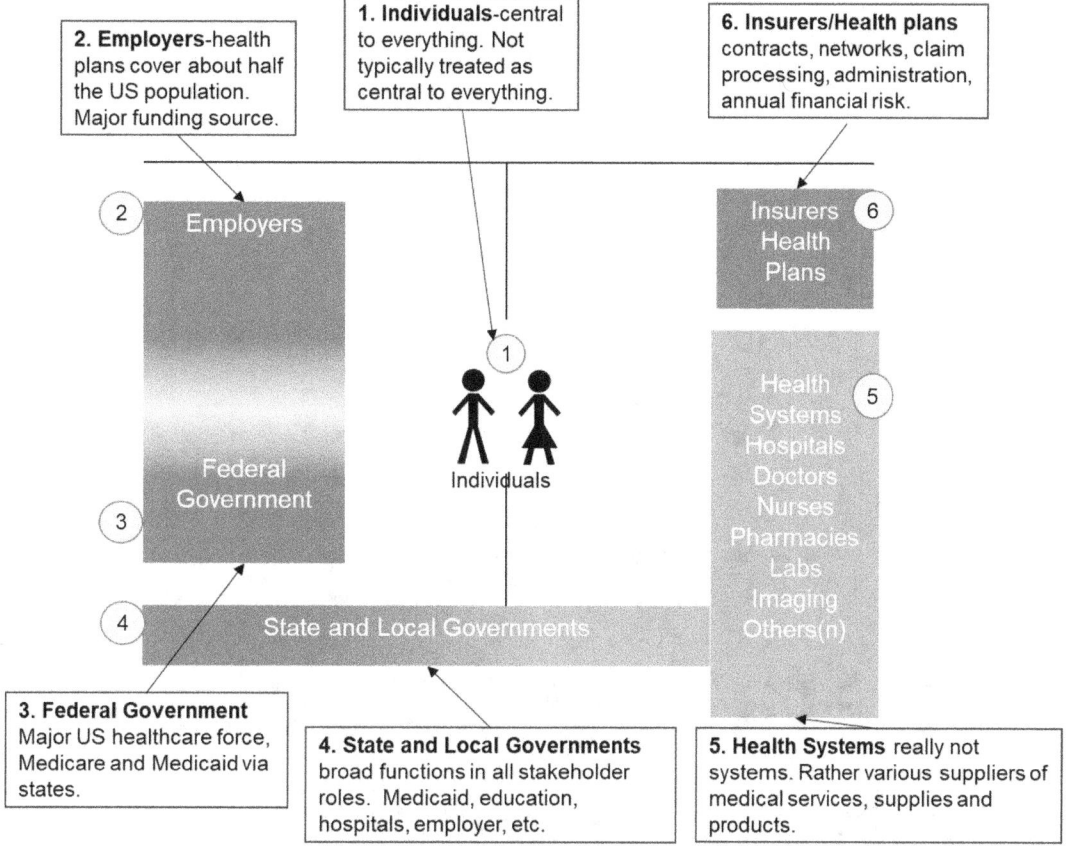

Operationally, here's how the system works:

1. **Individuals** are the ultimate consumers, customers, patients, living without much health system connection.
2. They are covered by a **health plan** funded by employer plans or governments.
3. They seek treatment in multiple locations and entry points when illness or injury occurs. This moment, however, is currently in significant change. Examples are primary care doctor changes through concierge, closing practices, advancing Nurse Practitioners and Physician Assistants, retailers entering primary care, and many more.
4. At the end of the day? The local hospital Emergency Room.
5. The episode progresses through whatever services are needed for the patient to return to health.
6. **Health systems** submit claims to the patient's insurer, health plan, or administrator.
7. The **insurer, health plan**, or **administrator adjudicates** the claim based on the various contracts with the healthcare providers.
8. Life goes on; return to #1.

This view makes it easy to see how the 'system' is not really a system. Rather, it is a fragmented health/medical treatment response to patients who seek their services.

Section 2:
Healthcare's operating structure on its foundation

SDOH plus other life and living elements

Social determinants of health (SDOH), health equity, and numerous community needs and resources are major 2023 focuses. That's appropriate. We need places to live, things to eat, knowledge, work, society, things to do, and more.

Dr. Berwick skillfully pinpoints that the health system is not the current source for resolving those community elements.

2023 and the near-term future are set for a constructive, peaceful revolution: blending day-to-day elements with medical treatment. Diagrams 4–7 outline the need for improved ways of addressing SDOH, other factors, and healthcare issues.

Diagram 4: Life and living, SDOH, etc. – the very basics

- Life
- Living
- Food
- Housing
- Jobs
- Security
- Social Life
- Education
- Transportation
- Family
- Play
- Fun
- Life at it fullest
- Add your own list entries

These are life's basics and the foundation of every community: housing, water, waste disposal, roads, transportation, schools/education, social programs, safety, fire protection, etc.

Local communities are responsible for providing the environment and resources for day-to-day living. They are also responsible for providing healthcare: medical treatment that restores health when lost or impaired by sickness or injury.

Diagram 5: Illness, injury, acute care, and chronic care all lead back to the life and living list

> - Patient, is not on the life/living list
> - When treatment is needed, we want the best, now, cost is no object
> - Healthcare restores us to the life list

Diagram 6: A synthesis of the healthcare problem

Diagram 6 represents, proportionally, life as it occurs. On the left are all the daily details of living. On the right are healthcare and medical treatment – that which restores lost or impaired health.

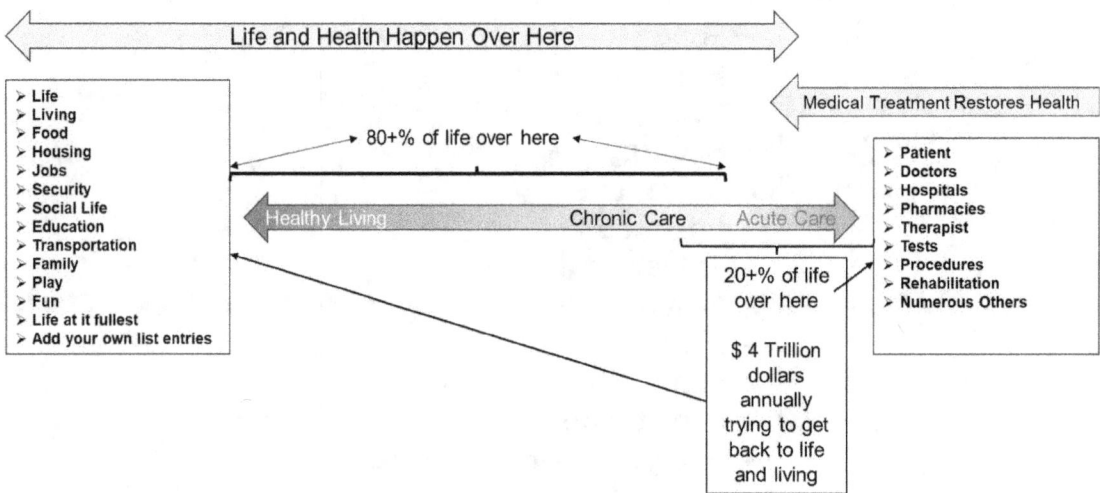

When the problem is outlined like that, it seems very obvious.

- We want to be healthy and live vibrant lives.
- We generally know what doing that takes.
- There's a lot of personal responsibility (a whole additional subject).
- When health is lost or compromised, we turn to our health systems to fix it immediately and without regard to cost.
- Who designed a role description for health systems to make life good for us?

Diagram 6 falls right into the Real Population Health™ sweet spot:

- There is no "person" in that middle role for individuals and populations.
- There is no coordinated information to support a person who wants or tries to fill that gap.
- Real Population Health™ improves health, healthcare, and costs. MUST fill that gap with information and dedicated, trained, and led people.

Diagram 7: How US healthcare is, operates, and feels

The US healthcare foundation lays solid groundwork for what happens next based on life apportionment. Diagram 7 shows how it really works and feels.

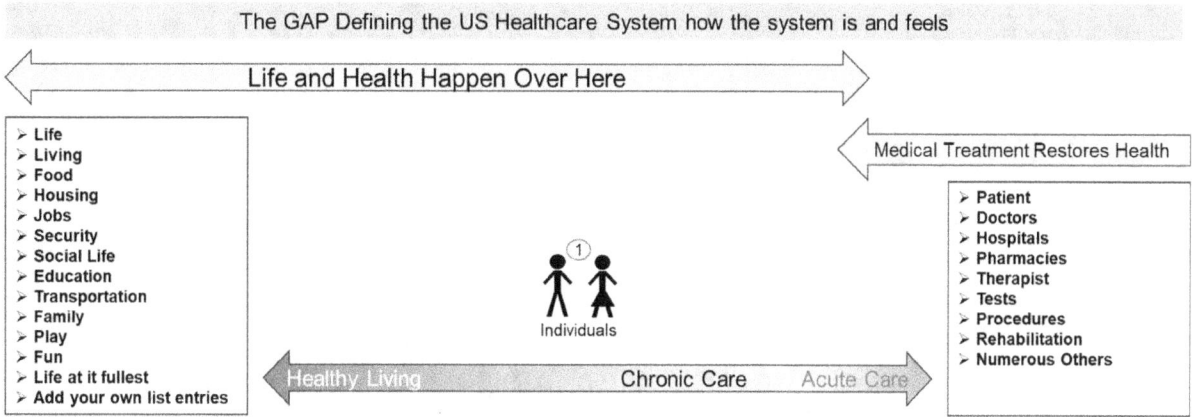

This is an excellent representation of our US healthcare system.

On the left: life and living, day-to-day, details, school, work, movement, activities, decisions, results, successes, and failures. Many acronyms (SDOH, HE, ADL, IADL), medical records, etc.

On the right: the health system whose role is restoring health when it's lost or compromised.

There are multiple reasons for the isolation of left from right.

    a. Third-party payment: individuals and consumers don't pay for the bulk of claim costs.
    b. As individuals, we want to find someone who can make us better.
    c. There is clear bifurcation amongst the six stakeholders, especially money and treatment.
    d. In the $4 trillion annual spend, there's very little for actual health improvement or effective medical resource use.
    e. In 2023, a lot is spent on billing, collection, and disputes over what's covered and what's not, along with what's appropriate or not.
    f. And maybe one of the biggest challenges.
        i. Conflicts across what's local, regional, and national. To a great extent, healthcare is local. However, financing healthcare is BIG national and regional money.
        ii. Healthcare's local nature in three very different categories:
            1) Metropolitan
            2) Urban
            3) Rural

Section 3:

"What the heck" is happening with Healthcare 2023?

That's why you invited us to the party!!

It's chaos – its own brand of US healthcare chaos. Here are four current examples.

1. At the beginning of this book, "American health systems must <u>transform radically</u>."
2. Becker's Healthcare: "Big companies crave healthcare savvy CEO's."
3. Kaiser Permanente: "Protests in LA, stress, working conditions."
4. Advisory Board: "600 rural hospitals at risk of closing."

The HMO Act of 1973 fixed it, right? Fifty years and millions of dollars spent/invested – so much for that **<u>one big move</u>** resolving all problems.

Integrating and aligning financial incentives for local hospitals/health systems to improve health, healthcare, and cost. Right?

I'm not too jaded in life. I have helped form and operate two provider-sponsored HMOs in the 80s and 90s. They worked. Aligned incentives. Collaborative and merged hospital-physician organizations. Hit the triple aim of better health, healthcare, and cost. One was sold to the highest bidder. One went broke due to underpricing and leadership fraud.

My healthcare bottom line is:

1. **Continued healthcare chaos:** this is understandable if you accept the notion of totally unlimited healthcare demand.
2. **Status quo:** so much money is on the table for the status quo. It's EVERYWHERE.

Wow, I'm re-reading that. That's so negative. Can't paint a rosy picture.

So why fight on, Harry? Two reasons:

1. **Older people in America** (I'm one of them): there are about 60 million over age 65 in the US today. That number will grow to about 90 million in 2060. Many/most are totally unprepared for old age for housing, income, food, SDOH, and healthcare.
2. **A simple healthcare solution that works**: over the past 50 years, I've practiced a simple healthcare structure and process that really works. Done it for various healthcare stakeholders (employers, health systems, TPA's, and some governments). It's a simple concept: just data, information, and relationships.

There's actually a **third reason** to fight on. As a Texan cowboy wanna-be, I have a strong tie to small towns – the people who live there and feed us. A hundred hospitals in Texas are on the verge of folding, owned by their local government. There are strained local resources to take care of older and end-of-life care (EOL) for those people. The data, information, and relationship model can be a big game changer for many rural people.

The realistic "What the Heck" bottom line? Sorry, it's status quo, chaos, chasing profits in non-profit worlds, consolidation, closings, etc. A tough but noble battleground.

So, the real answer and bottom line to "What the Heck" is going on with US healthcare?

1. It is broken. That's not news. We're not piling on additional proofs or details.

2. Some simple things can be done within the current healthcare foundations, structures, and operations.

3. There are six defined healthcare stakeholders, and leadership can come from any of them. There's an individual limitation due to third-party payment. In other direct-pay professions and businesses, individual consumers vote every day with their feet and pocketbooks. Healthcare is not the model. Somebody else pays.

4. Real payers, with real long-term risks (employers and governments) will step up and force the alignment of financial models to improve health, healthcare, and cost.

5. Leadership can come from any of the stakeholders. And collaboration amongst stakeholders enhances the process.

6. Local is where healthcare happens. Leadership amongst the stakeholders at the local level becomes the most powerful.

7. There is a model that is available now, within our grasp.

    a. **Local populations:** small, a few, a few hundred, a few thousand, rolling up into cities and metropolises.
    b. **Information** spanning SDOH, critical health improvement, and treatment information
    c. **Professionals**, Personal Health Nurses, Primary Care Doctors, NPs, and PAs with long-term ongoing relationships with the individuals within their populations.

These local populations can connect through today's technology with Academic Medical Centers. Forty-eight of 52 states have Academic Medical Centers that can integrally serve:

  a. Local communities, small communities where SDOH and daily life go on.
  b. Local resources that match local populations. See 7a above and population sizes in Section 5.
  c. Local professionals take care of the routine community needs.
  d. Complex conditions go straight to the AMC, along with key information.
  e. Returning home is smooth, safe, and effective through technological connectivity.
  f. Local resources match the population, focus on SDOH and local service, and directly access the resources of AMC with VERY individual customer-friendly support in, out, and through episodes of care with compassionate efficient EOL care.

More on that later in the book.

Section 4:
A proven healthcare improvement process

The proven healthcare improvement consists of data/information captured, stored, and accessed securely and a personal relationship with a qualified, trained healthcare professional.

1. **Creative use of data and information** that are individual and population specific.

2. **Creating and operating "relationships"** amongst individuals, their information, for health improvement/treatment, and other resources.

Regardless of healthcare's foundation, structure, and operations, any of the six healthcare stakeholders an implement the proven improvement.

Diagram 8: The proven improvement diagram and details

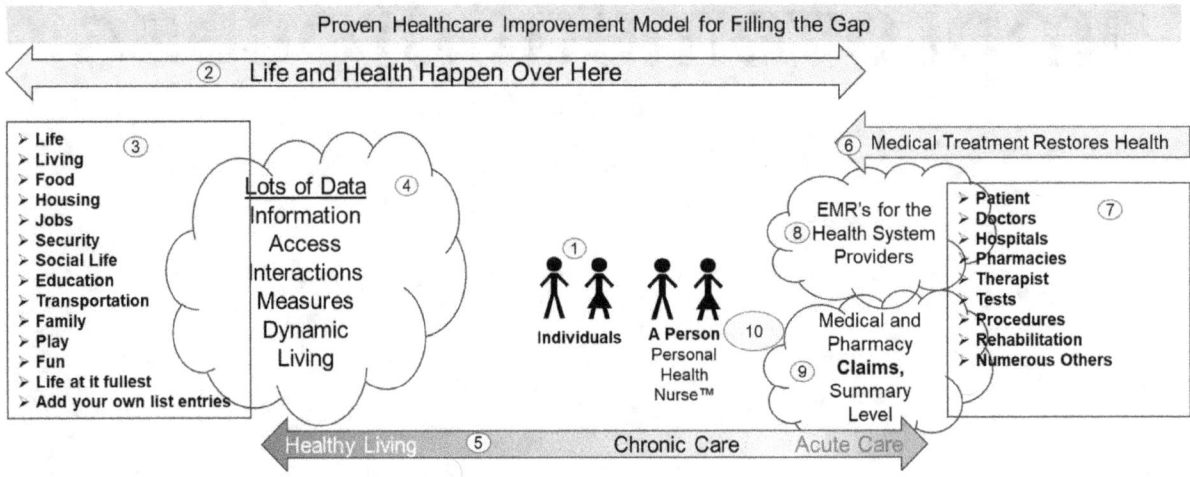

Details of the process follow on the next page.

Here are additional details for Diagram 8.

1. Individual clients are the core, the focus, and the reason for operating.

2. We spend most of our lives in the healthy domain. Even with chronic conditions, with excellent coordination, we live the best lives we can with our conditions.

3. A partial list of life, SDOH, and living activities provides a sample for consideration.

4. Data: the model becomes a bit more complicated at this point. The complication grows, then comes into focus with the addition of # 10, the health professional with an ongoing relationship with the individual.

5. That two-pointed arrow shows that we have conditions that arise, needing chronic and acute care. A typical population in any given year will only have 10–20% of the population in the high-risk high-cost categories. Individuals will migrate through those categories.

6. Medical treatment and episodes of care occur as needed by individuals.

7. Healthcare (medical treatment) is delivered by doctors, nurses, technicians, pharmacist, various therapists, technicians, and hosts of others.

   In a fee-for-service environment, those providers using their Electronic Medical Records (EMR) submit their bills with the required information to be reimbursed by the appropriate insurer or health plan.

   Most providers will use a centralized EMR for data management in a capitated environment.

8. The various EMRs, through billing systems or Health Information Networks, submit and usually also post payments.

9. A unique, extremely valuable resource is the population claim data provided by the insurer or health plan. This summarizes all the transactions for each person that rolls up to the population, providing key information distilled from the EMRs.

10. The final piece, whose value is significantly positively leveraged by elements 1–9. More will be said about this. A Population Operating Manual is available for maximum detail.

This improvement works for all healthcare stakeholders.

It also works in all types of financing methods. The nuances of structure and operation change to fit the circumstances.

Diagram 9: How the improvement model fits within the financial foundation

Here I am repeating an earlier US healthcare foundation diagram in financial reporting form.

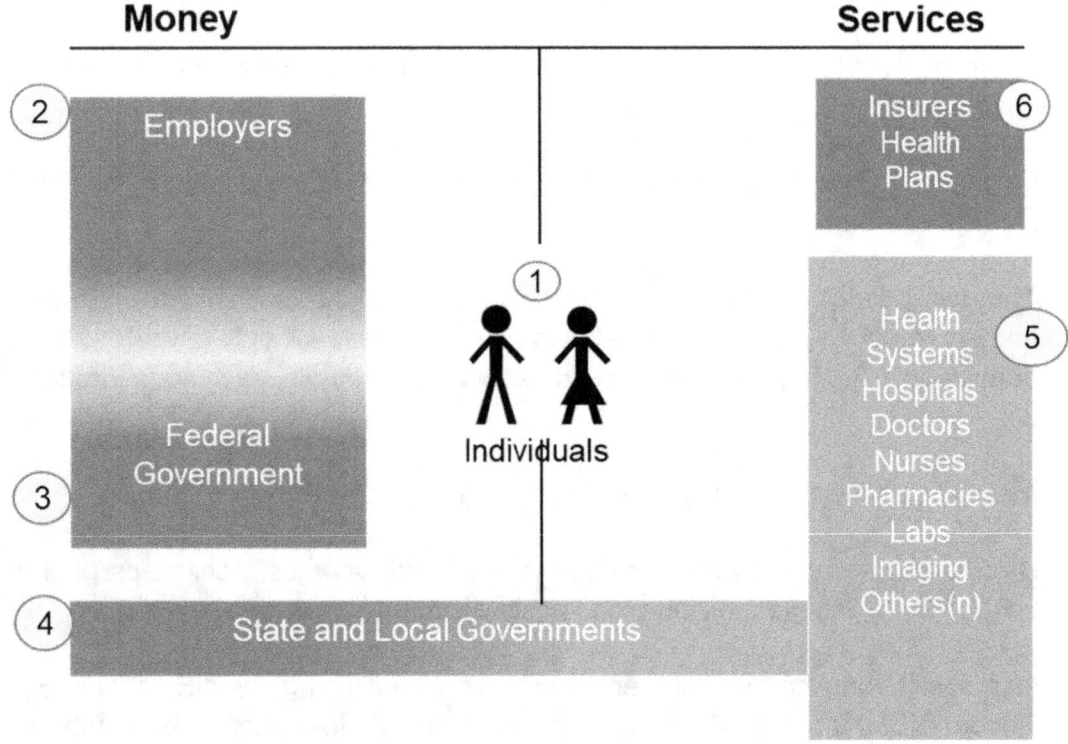

This diagram shows the plight of individuals caught in how healthcare is financed and administered.

The other side of that coin is how individuals are caught in life circumstances.

Diagram 10: Major gap among life, living, treatment, and resources

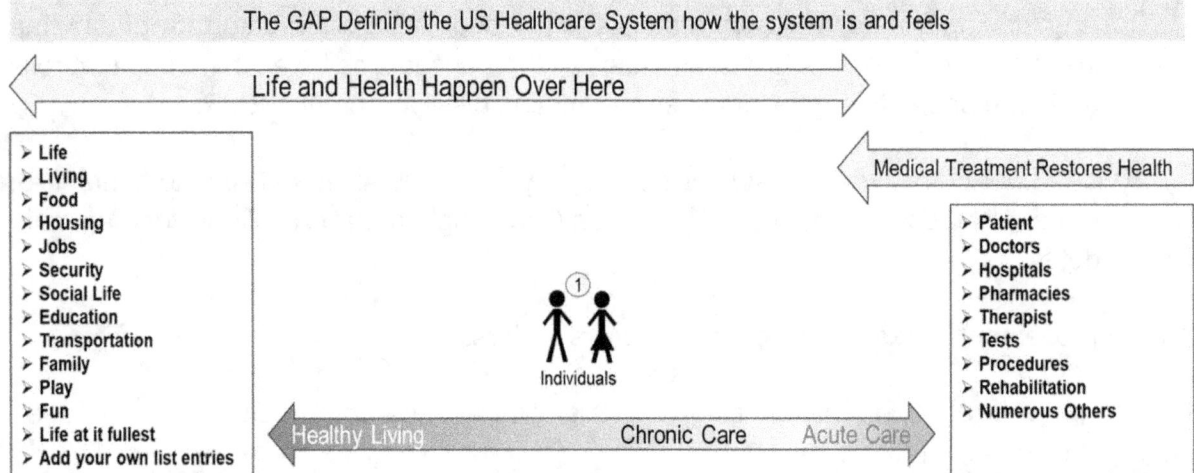

By addressing their life circumstances and helping individuals achieve their best health and healthcare, the improvement also fits within the financial foundation of the US healthcare system.

Diagram 11: A proven structure and operation for improved healthcare results

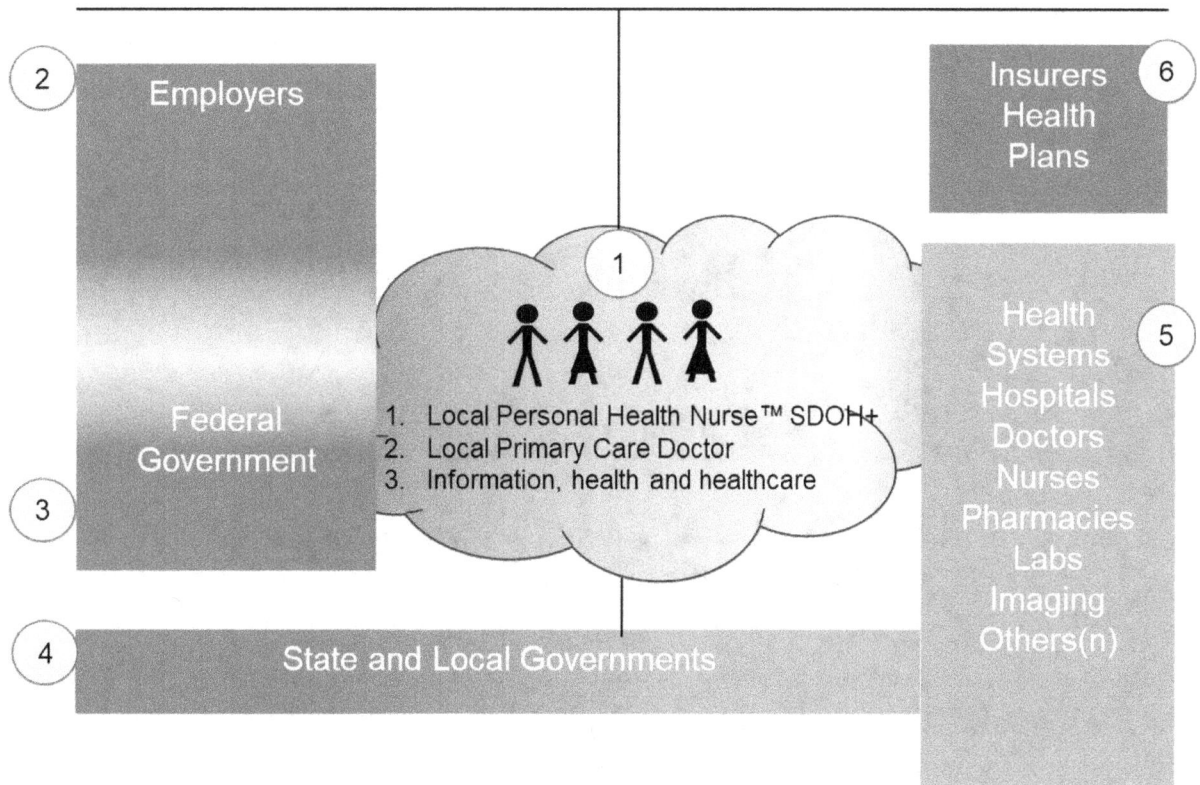

Individuals have "a person." How novel. No matter how automated we get, other professions and businesses still have "people" to help when all else fails. Granted, we must go through many phone trees, computer clicks, etc. But to get what we want, we ultimately need a fellow human.

This is not quite the case in healthcare, maybe our most complicated and important activities. Each element of healthcare takes care of its part. The lab knows its part. Doctors know their part. Etc., etc.

Oh, you say, "My health system has a 'patient portal.'" Yup, they all do. But who really knows me, my conditions, and my circumstances?

In 2022–2023, our family has two daughters who have had four inpatient procedures. They were done in the best hospital and health system. But, things as simple as transportation, transition to physical therapy, etc. – anyone who uses the system knows EXACTLY what I mean.

Section 5:
A template for US healthcare

The basic building blocks for the template

1. We are in healthcare chaos primarily due to individual consumers being ignored, abused, and left alone. That position starts with the executive summary and continues throughout. Resolving and improving that fatal flaw is fundamental and critical.
2. A proven improvement model that addresses problem #1 is in place and can be replicated.
3. The proven model is not capital or fixed-cost intensive.
4. Any of the six healthcare stakeholders can lead and drive the model.
5. We need data management for healthcare services, especially focused on better health, personal habits supporting better health, and proper resources when needed.
6. The individual interface should be local, in the neighborhood health professional. Our recurring bias is Personal Health Nurses™ for numerous reasons. That doesn't rule out other professions or qualifications as long as long-term relationships are formed, cultivated, and producing results.
7. There should be a preferred acute care hospital. No special arrangements are needed to initiate the plan.
8. There should also be a tertiary care hospital for complicated conditions. Frequently, that naturally is that state's Academic Medical Center.

The sustainable end game

1. **Identified population.** Designation will most likely be geographic. Neighborhood, zip code, town, county, hospital service area, employer group, etc. The population will need to have somewhat common healthcare preferences.
2. **Committed payer.** The Federal Government and employers are the natural ultimate payers. However, that does not preclude state and local governments, health systems, or insurers/health plans.
3. **Committed leader.** A leader from a stakeholder category.
4. **Enrolled membership.** Individuals who are enrolled execute necessary forms and releases. The sponsoring organization controls membership.
5. **Data Management System.** The system must support the operation along with reporting and data analytics. MyHealthPlace® is our unique owned resource for that function.
6. **Operations Manuals.** Guiding the operations of the population.
7. **Client contact professionals.** Our recurring preference is Personal Health Nurses™ who are specialized RNs.
8. **Local Primary Care Doctors.** They integrate with the overall strategy.
9. **The mix of professionals.** Amongst NPs, PAs, etc., can fit well into the structure.

A functional operation

1. **Population or populations.** The surprise here will be the small size. Expect populations of about 100–400 at the core.

   Considerations for population size:
   a. The population's annual healthcare costs range from $1.5 million to $5 million. Sizable business.
   b. Medicare's population-nurse ratio averages 1:100, and the monthly cost is about $125.
   c. Commercial's population-nurse ratio averages 1:400, and the monthly cost is about $40.
   d. Primary care doctors should average 1:1,000 or as high as 1:5,000, based on age, conditions, and working relationships with nurses.

2. Nurses generally work from home with a member meeting place convenient to the members and the nurse.

3. Doctors generally work in a traditional clinic environment.

4. Pharmacies typically are the ones favored by members.

5. General acute care hospitals will be the ones favored by members.

6. The member, nurse, and primary care doctor will use the appropriate Academic Medical Center for complex care. The pathways into the system and discharge back to home or other facilities are closely monitored and guided by the local nurse and primary care doctor.

At this point, it is important to note the use of a consumer-friendly information system. Several components are mission-critical, such as medical history, SDOH, ADLs, health improvement scores, etc. But, the key is the value of chronology between the member and the nurse.

Those data are securely transmittable and can follow the member during their episode as a patient. Chronological samples are shown below.

Diagram 12: Sample nurse/client interactions over time

Corporate

Date	Interactions
16-Feb	Member notified this nurse that member is in the ER for lightheadedness. Member did not feel well. This RN assess member's symptoms and advise member to ask for lab results and imaging result when done.
25-Feb	Following up with member, member states that member feels better. Member sent home with probiotic for Colitis. Member states that member still has symptoms intermittently.
2-Mar	Member still has symptoms of flushing, numbness, epigastric pain, dizziness episodically, it comes and goes. Appointments are made with GI and Cardiologist.
30-Mar	This RN advised ER, admitted Pacemaker installed
10-Apr	Member is back to work on light duty. Member reports he is doing well, feeling some depression due to recent health changes. Member is thankful of being alive. Member is working on his recovery. Member is offered resources and counseling. Will continue to follow up with member.
	14 face to face interactions February 16, 2023 through May 8, 2023

Medicare

Date	Interactions
12/28/2021	member is besides himself. he was out of Prozac for the past week and sat home over Christmas with a pounding headache, no medications and frozen waffles to eat by himself. States he cried a lot. He has requested paperwork from his Dr. for M on W, as have we at Wecare and the paperwork has never been received at M on W. The documentation of calls and faxes is almost endless. He has requested a shower chair from Tidemark, and it has been over 4 months, and the chair has still not arrived. He lives on $250/ food stamps and $79/ month. he was just told that is suspended and he does not know why. his daughter is in the hospital for cancer and is having a 3rd surgery this week because they found more tumors. Member states he will need new housing arrangements because his living situation is temporary. he does not want to be at The Capital Inn in Dover. He says he witnessed people get shot there. Information provided to traveling NP/ primary care option if he wants to investigate other PCP options. Referral request sent to Comfort care because he has Medicaid/Tidemark. Hopeful Ms. XXXXXX at Comfort care will give us an avenue.
1/1/2022	Initiated LTC paperwork through DELAWARE HEALTH AND SOCIAL SERVICES DIVISION OF MEDICAID & MEDICAL ASSISTANCE. Application will need to be signed by member. Once it is received to our office via email, it will be forwarded to MrXXXXXX, via email. Mr. XXXXXX has a multitude of concerns, and states he is very confused alot of the time. Says he can only buy cold food with food stamps, he is not alloowed to buy a rotiserri chicken, or warm coup. Says he has not had a warm meal in months. It seems that Meals on Wheels may be initiated as of this up and coming Monday, we will see! Is considering to change doctors, but will wait until after this application is processed. Daughter is awaiting another surgical procedure
	54 intervening interactions
10/24/2022	I spoke to Mr. XXXXXXXX this morning. He stated he is now in Wilmington, safe and healthy. He expressed his gratitude for WeCare.

A 'per member per month' example of resource realignment

Populations that implement the proven improved healthcare process are experiencing and have experienced PMPM reductions and reallocations of expenses similar to the table below.

Diagram 13: Sample per member per month (PMPM) allocation

Proven Improved Process Healthcare PMPM							
Assumptions	Traditional			Real Population Health		Variation	
PMPM	$ 1,200		PMPM	$ 1,080	90%	$ (120)	-10%
Administration	$ 108	9%	Administration	$ 54	5%	$ (54)	-50%
Risk	$ 108	9%	Risk	$ 54	5%	$ (54)	-50%
Adm/Risk Sub-Total	$ 216	18%		$ 108	10%	$ (108)	-50%
Inpatient	$ 348	29%	Inpatient	$ 313	29%	$ (35)	-10%
Outpatient	$ 240	20%	Outpatient	$ 216	20%	$ (24)	-10%
Specialists	$ 228	19%	Specialists	$ 205	19%	$ (23)	-10%
Primary Care	$ 48	4%	Primary Care	$ 65	6%	$ 17	35%
Personal Health Nurse	$ -	0	Personal Health Nurse	$ 65	6%	$ 65	54%
Pharmacy	$ 120	10%	Pharmacy	$ 108	10%	$ (12)	-1%
Medical Sub-total	$ 984	100%		$ 972	100%	$ (120)	
Total	$ 1,200			$ 1,080		$ (120)	10%

Input profile
1. General blended population Medicare, Medicaid, Employer
2. 1 Nurse per 200 members, 400 for Employer, 100 for High-risk aging
3. 1 Primary care doctor per 5-10 nurses and 1,000-2,000 members
4. Administration and risk moved from admininstrative oversight to consumer friendly health professionals

Something that MUST be said is that local hospitals resist "taking risk," primarily meaning taking the annual financial risk for a population. Meanwhile, three things: 1) hospitals are typically one of the biggest businesses in any town, 2) ACA makes every employer in that town 100% at annual financial risk for their employee population, and 3) especially in small towns, the employers' main risk is what migrates out of that town. It's a real recipe for disaster for that community.

Summary

We started by discussing US healthcare's brokenness. We identified that individuals are caught between **enormous** financial/administrative and data/information gaps. Healthcare individuals/consumers/patients have no cohesive, available, customer-friendly place to turn outside their medical treatment episodes.

We alluded to the probable reality that the problems will compound as the US population ages.

And amidst all that, there is a fairly simple approach of utilizing data in expanded ways and providing ongoing customer-friendly relationships to individuals.

May we make huge dents in the status quo.

Rural Healthcare Appendix

The rural US presents perfect conditions for healthcare improvement through innovation.

Widely dispersed population, large (46 million), over huge territory, small communities of people, traditional healthcare under duress.

Rural US Healthcare's position and circumstances create excellent environments for innovation and improvement. Those innovations might establish useful templates for managing large urban populations segmented into manageable population subsets.

The *What the Heck* book diagrams outline current and possible healthcare delivery models. Those diagrams resolve into the proven healthcare improvement model, diagrammed below and uniquely applicable to rural US.

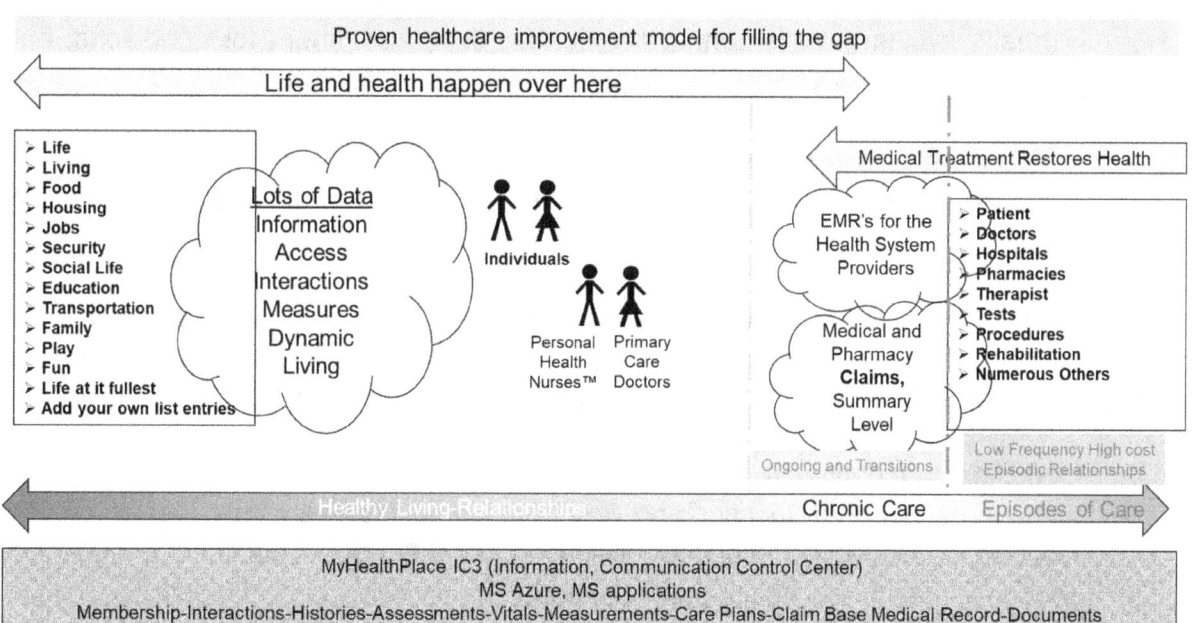

The proven working model:

1. **Individuals comprise the model's center** and are central to their health and healthcare. That immediately flips the healthcare focus 180 degrees.

   Historic population health is all about conditions, "all the diabetes over here, cardiac over there," then we see how well we treat those groups.

   That's not how personal/real population health works. My ailments are not a group experience. They are one on one, one at a time. This is especially pertinent to rural US.

2. **The individual has relationships** with a Personal Health Nurse™ plus, a Primary Care Doctor, a Nurse Practitioner, a Physician Assistant, and other emerging primary medical care professionals. The person and their team focus on:

   a. Best possible health in the broad definition of Social Determinants of Health (SDOH). Plus, senior-specific: Activities of Daily Living (ADLs), and Instrumental Activities of Daily Living (IADLs). Across all the individuals within their population, the "medical intake data" is secure, accessible, and acceptable values such as vitals, assessments, medical history, care plans, etc.

   b. Best possible treatment when conditions occur, best quality, best price.
      i. Local based on local services and resources.
      ii. Regional health systems in larger accessible communities.
      iii. Tertiary specialty health systems for complex care.

   c. In all circumstances, for all individuals in the local population, intense focus applies to movement into, out of and within various health systems. A key US health system flaw is connecting healthy living, treatment for conditions, and returning to active living.

   Special attention to these navigations and supporting information dramatically improves rural citizens' lives. End-of-life planning and actual practice play critical real population roles.

For numerous reasons, rural US uniquely benefits by capitalizing on the model diagramed and described above. Rural US faces unique risks, challenges, and equally unique opportunities for implementing and operating Real Population Health™ that is each community unique.

- Populations are definable.
- Cultures are unique by location and vary from typical urban settings.
- Health resources vary from extremely limited to good to excellent.
- Frequently, health and health quality already benefit from local relationships.
- Implementing the structures and operations outlined in Real Population Health™ can dramatically enhance health and healthcare in rural communities.

Location circumstances and resources preclude specific prescriptive directions. Rather, the next few pages outline strategic contexts that will help local leaders advance their best community health, healthcare, and cost.

A summary of US community numbers and percentages reveals dramatic rural statistics.

84.14% of communities under 10,000 population? That dramatically underscores problems, challenges, and opportunities.

US Communties by Population		
Community Population	Number in US	Percent
>1,000,000	10	0.05%
500,000-999,000	27	0.14%
250,000-499,000	52	0.27%
100,000-249,000	225	1.15%
50,000-99,999	466	2.39%
>50,000 Subtotal	780	4.00%
25,000-49,999	741	3.80%
10,000-24,999	1,572	8.06%
Under 10,000	16,410	84.14%
<50,000 Subtotal	18,723	96.00%
Total	**19,503**	100%

This data leads to repeating "why rural populations" in the appendix introduction.

3. 97% of US land is rural.

4. 15% of the population (46 million) live in rural US, larger than any single US state.

5. 90% of the food we eat is grown in rural US.

6. 17.5% of the population in rural areas are older than 65, compared to 13.8% urban areas, or a 27% higher rate.

7. 42% "of Americans would like to live in rural areas or towns."

8. Approximately 2,000 hospitals, 30% "teetering on the edge of closure."

A rural population summary statement:

> A large US population by size and percent
> live in rural US.
> 84% of our communities have a population of 50,000 or less.
> The ideal locations to build health, healthcare, and cost
> from the ground up.

Section 5 of the *What the Heck* book provides a template for building local healthcare from the ground up, small populations at a time. Intentionally not prescriptive. But it provides structures and possibilities. Below is an outline of Section 5:

1. **Identified population** – natural to rural US.
2. **Committed payer** – Governments (Federal, State, Local) and employers.
3. **Committed leaders** – can be from any stakeholder perspective. Passionate and committed to change.
4. **Enrolled membership** – integral membership management.
5. **Data management system** – such as IC3/MyHealthPlace®.
6. **Operating Manuals** – that fit the community.
7. **Client contact professionals** – a continued preference for Personal Health Nurses™ collaborating with local, regional, and centers of excellence primary care.
8. **Local Primary Care Doctors** – in communities large enough to support them. Excellent opportunities for telehealth with local Personal Health Nurses™.

EVERY rural community creates its own place in the world. From a very small and far from any larger town to a mid-sized town close to urban areas. There is no "one-size fits all." However, building from the ground up with populations of 100+/- with:

- Personal Health Nurses™.
- Solid, accurate, secure, individual health and healthcare information.
- Connections with Primary Care.
- Connections with health systems centers of excellence.
- Tied to individual members with advancing technologies.

Rural US has the opportunity to create new and better pathways to better health, healthcare, and cost.

One key point. Governments, especially the Federal Government, will play key roles in rural solutions. State and local governments will also be key players. Their roles will include various non-traditional activities, probably including providing local health care professionals.

The *Real Population Health Operating Manual 2022* is relevant and available on Amazon/Kindle for those wanting more.

Rural Summary

1. Rural US – very challenging for numerous reasons.
2. We must pursue something different.
3. Layering urban top-down solutions onto rural US destined to fail.
4. Individual focus, relationship-driven, information-supported local healthcare with rational out-of-area referrals work and can light the way for the nation.

Sources from the appendix introductory page

1. Land percentage 97%: https://www.americanprogress.org/article/redefining-rural-america/
2. Population 15% or 46 million people: https://www.cdc.gov/ruralhealth/about.html
3. Food 90%: https://www.eatright.org/food/planning/food-security-and-sustainability/where-does-our-food-come_from#:~:text=In%20fact%2C%20in%202016%2C%20close,soybeans%2C%20milk%20and%20other%20dairy
4. Rural population over age 65 is 17.5%, 27% higher than: https://www.ncbi.nlm.nih.gov/pmc/articles/PMC9644394/#:~:text=Furthermore%2C%20although%20only%2015%25%20of,of%20urban%20populations%20%5B5%5D.
5. 42% want to live in rural areas: https://www.aei.org/politics-and-public-opinion/a-real-rural-future/#:~:text=The%20lion's%20share%20of%20Americans,who%20would%20prefer%20suburban%20areas.
6. 600 or 30% of rural hospitals "are teetering on the edge of closure": https://www.usnews.com/news/health-news/articles/2023-01-16/hundreds-of-hospitals-could-close-across-rural-america
7. Cities and towns by population size: https://www.statista.com/statistics/241695/number-of-us-cities-towns-villages-by-population-size/
8. PCPs: https://www.globenewswire.com/en/news-release/2023/03/15/2627511/28124/en/U-S-Primary-Care-Physicians-Market-Report-2023-Affordable-Care-Act-Continues-to-Bolster-Sector.html#:~:text=According%20to%20Kaiser%20Family%20Foundation,accounting%20for%20205%2C285%20active%20physicians.
9. NPs: https://www.aanp.org/about/all-about-nps/np-fact-sheet
10. PAs: https://www.aapa.org/about/what-is-a-pa/#:~:text=There%20are%20more%20than%20168%2C300,workplace%20clinics%2C%20and%20correctional%20institutions.
11. Working definitions for rural, urban, etc.: https://nces.ed.gov/programs/edge/docs/locale_classifications.pdf

About the Author

Harry Spring is a lifetime healthcare professional practicing various innovative ways to improve health and pursue Real Population Health™.

"Individuals living their best possible lives, including:

- Best health
- Best healthcare
- Reasonable cost."

RealPHN and various collaborating organizations provide services to any of the six healthcare stakeholders, from strategy to implementation, training, and operation.

The services always return to:

1. Filling healthcare's missing piece with services through relationships, Personal Health Nurses™, and local Primary Care Doctors.

2. Supported by unique information deployment.

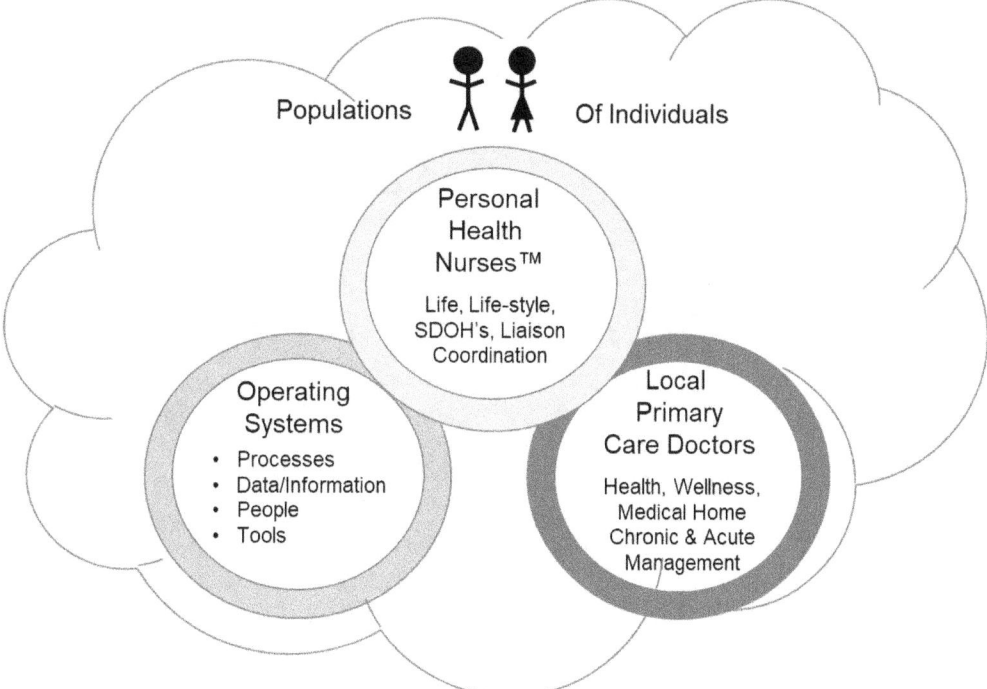

www.ingramcontent.com/pod-product-compliance
Lightning Source LLC
Chambersburg PA
CBHW062236220526
45471CB00009B/3505